국제 진료 영어

본 과제(결과물)는 교육과학기술부의 재원으로 한국연구재단의 지원을 받아 수행된 광역경제권 선도산업 인재양성사업의 연구 결과입니다.

국제 진료 영어

| 이종호 · 안무업 지음 |

小花

머리말

우리말로 해도 진료는 어렵습니다. 무엇보다 소중한 인명과 관련된 일이며 때로는 촌각을 다투는 위급한 상황도 발생하기 때문입니다. 제한된 시간 내에 정확한 진단을 위해서는 간결하면서도 체계적인 소통이 필수적인데, 국경을 넘나드는 글로벌 시대의 진료에서는 언어의 차이에서 비롯되는 어려움까지 가중되고 있습니다. 실제로 2010년 기준, 한국에 거주하는 외국인 수가 100만 명이 넘으며 유학을 가는 한국인 수도 매년 증가하고 있습니다. 그간 공적으로나 사적으로나 영어교육에 막대한 자원이 투자되었지만, 진료 영어는 여전히 생소하며, 평소에 익숙하던 영어도 의료 현장에서는 바로 적용하기 힘든 경우가 빈번합니다.

이 책은, 어느 언어든 반복해서 필요한 상황별로 학습한다면 어려운 상황에 효과적으로 대비할 수 있다는 점을 바탕으로, 의사국가고시 실기시험인 OSCE, CPX에 필요한 환자와의 진료 대화를 영어로 다루었습니다. OSCE는 병력 청취, 신체 진찰, 검사술기, 치료 및 처치기술 중 단일항목에 대해 세부적으로 의과 진료를 수행하는 능력을 평가하며, CPX에서는 OSCE 모든 항목에 대해 모의 환자를 상대로 의사와 환자의 관계를 평가합니다. 두 시험에서 공통 항목으로 다루어지는, 의사의 진료 특성상 응급 상황은 항상 발생하므로 반복, 훈련함으로써 주어진 상황에 반사적으로 대답이 나올 수 있어야 합니다.

증상 카테고리, 상황별로 대화를 나누어 질문과 그에 응하는 대답을 순서대로 나열함으로써 진료 영어에 좀 더 쉽게 접근하려 하였습니다. 증상별로 주요 감별진단을 숙지하고, 병력 청취 시에 증상의 시작, 위치부터 시작해서 동반 증상 등을 묻는 세부적인 부분으로 점차 들어가는 방식을 취했습니다. 이 책을 통해 환자의 특징적인 병력의 파악에 필요한 지문을 폭넓게 익힘으로써 외국인 환자를 접하는 상황에서 능숙히 대처할 수 있기를 바랍니다. 앞서 언급했듯이, 가능한 다양한 상황을 예상하고 준비한다면 급변하는 국제화 시대에 더욱 준비된 의사가 될 수 있을 것입니다.

정부에서도 한국 사회의 신(新)성장 동력으로 의료관광 사업을 주목하고 있는 현 시점에, 국제 진료 영어를 미리 접하고 익힘으로써 수월하게 더 넓은 세계로 도약하기를 바랍니다.

2011년 3월
저자 이종호, 안무업

차례

6. Joint and Limb Pain

7. Low Back Pain

8. Dizziness

9. Confusion and Memory Loss

12. Amenorrhea

13. Vaginal Bleeding

14. Vaginal Discharge

15. Child with Fever

16. Weight Loss and Gain

17. Upper GI Bleeding

18. Blood in Stool

19. Constipation and Diarrhea

1. Headache

Differential Diagnosis

Migraine	Despite lacking aura, the patient's presentation is classic for this diagnosis.
Tension headache	Bilateral and squeezing Lasts from hours to days and gets worse as the day progress.
Depression	Worse on arising in the morning
Pseudotumor cerebri	Focal headache Diplopia, visual symptoms
Cluster headache	Unilateral periorbital pain, often accompanied by ipsilateral nasal congestion, rhinorrhea, lacrimation, redness of the eye

Onset

- Question
  - When did it start?
  - Is pain always there or does it come and go?
- Answer
  - It started 3 hours ago after football practice.
  - Well, I think, it is continuous.

Location

- Question
  - Where do you feel the pain?
  - Please point to me exactly where the pain is?

• Answer
  - The entire left side of my head.
  - Bilateral side of my head.
  - It is here. (points to the whole right side of the head.)

Quality

• Question
  - What is the pain like?
  - Can you describe to me how it hurts?
  - Please describe your pain.

• Answer
  - Pounding and throbbing.
  - Sharp and pounding.

Severity

• Question
  - On a scale of 1 to 10, with 10 being the worst pain of your life, how would you rate your pain?
  - Have you ever waken up because of this pain?

• Answer
  - On a scale of 1 to 10, this is 10.
  - When I have the pain, it is 9 or 10, and prevents me from working.

Precipitating Factor

- Question
  - What brings the pain on?
  - Do you know what causes the pain to start?
- Answer
  - The stress of exams.
  - Important football games.

Aggravating and Alleviating Factor

- Question
  - Does anything make the pain better?
  - Have you tried anything to make this better?
  - Does anything make the pain worse?
- Answer
  - Closing my eyes and staying very still help.
  - I took 2 aspirin. However they didn't help.

Associated Symptoms

- Question
  - Have you noticed anything else besides your headache?
  - Do you feel nauseated?
  - Did you throw up?
  - Do you have warning that the headache is about to come?
- Answer
  - Sometimes I feel nauseated when I am in pain.
  - Yesterday I vomited for the first time.

- I vomited once and I still feel nauseated.
- Lights were flashing for about 20minutes before it started.

Past Medical History

- Question
  - Have you had similar pain before?
  - Have you had this problem or anything similar before?
  - Do you have any medical problems?
  - Have you been hospitalized before?
  - Have you had any surgeries before?
  - Are you taking any medications?
- Answer
  - Yes, in college I had a similar headache that was accompanied by nausea.
  - I have an episode of sinusitis four months ago, treated with amoxicillin. But the pain was different from the one I have now.

Social History

- Question
  - Do you smoke?
  - How many packs a day?
  - How long have you smoked?
  - Do you drink alcohol?
  - What do you drink?
  - How much do you drink per week?
  - Do you have a lot of stressful situations on your job?
  - Are you exposed to environmental hazard on your job?

- Answer
  - I smoke a pack per day.
  - I drink just a beer on Sundays.

Family History

- Question
  - Has anyone in your family ever had headache like this before?
- Answer
  - My mother and sister have migraines.

Dialogue

D: Good afternoon.

P: Good afternoon.

D: Let me introduce myself. My name is Dr. Choi. I'm a doctor working on this hospital. I'm going to ask you some questions and do a physical exam on you. After that I'll discuss with you what I think so far.

D: If you have any questions, I'd be happy to answer them anytime. What brings you here today?

P: I have a headache.

D: When did it start?

P: It started 2 hours ago.

D: Which part of your head is most painful?

P: My left side hurts.

D: Can you describe how the pain is like?

P: My head is throbbing and pounding.

D: What were you doing when the pain began?

P: I was at work, preparing for a meeting.

D: How severe is the pain? How much does the pain bother your normal activities?

P: I can withstand the pain, but can't concentrate well on my work.

D: When does the pain get worse, or better?

P: I don't know well, but I think it's related to stress.

D: Do you have any changes in your daily life or events that get you more stressed recently?

P: I have conferences more than usual, but it's not that much of a stress.

D: Are there any other symptoms beside the headache?

P: Before I get the headaches, my vision blurs, and I feel light-headed.

D: Are there any other symptoms?

P: I feel nauseated, but I didn't throw-up.

D: Did you get any head injuries recently?

P: No, I didn't.

D: Do you have a fever or any skin rash?

P: No, I don't.

D: Is it hard for you to move your neck?

P: No, my neck is fine.

D: Did these symptoms happen to you before?

P: The first time I had this pain is about a year ago. Ever since, it comes about twice a month.

D: When the pain starts, how long does it last?

P: It usually goes for roughly 8 hours.

D: Does the pills ease your pain?

P: The pain gets a little better, but doesn't go away.

D: Do you have any chronic diseases like diabetes or hypertension?

P: No, I don't have any of those diseases.

D: Do you take any medications regularly?

P: No, I take some pills when I have a headache.

D: Do you smoke? How much alcohol do you drink?

P: I don't smoke, and I drink one or two times a month.

D: How much alcohol do you drink once you do?

P: About half a bottle.

D: How much coffee or tea do you take in a day?

P: I always take my morning and afternoon coffee.

D: Does any of your relatives have similar symptoms?

P: My mother has headaches sometimes, but it's not severe as mine.

2. Loss of Consciousness

Differential Diagnosis

Convulsive syncope	Seizure like activity often occurs after syncope and is due to global cerebral hypoperfusion.
Vasovagal syncope	Occurs in the setting of emotional stress or pain and may be due to excessive vagal tone with resulting hypotension. Syncope is often heralded by nausea, sweating, tachycardia, pallor and feeling faint.
Cardiac arrhythmia	History of palpitation may indicate the presence of an underlying arrhythmia.
Seizure	Tonic-clonic seizures are often accompanied by tongue biting, incontinence, and prolonged confusion or drowsiness postictally.

Onset

- Question
  - When did it start?
  - When did you lose consciousness?
- Answer
  - It started three months ago.
  - This morning I was taking the groceries to the car with my wife when I suddenly fell down and blacked out.

Quality

- Question
  - Please describe your loss of consciousness.

- Answer
  - My wife told me that I did not respond to her for several minutes.

Precipitating Factor

- Question
  - Do you know what causes loss of consciousness?
- Answer
  - Well, I think just before I fell down, my heart started racing.

Associated Symptoms

- Question
  - Have you noticed anything else besides your Loss of consciousness?
- Answer
  - Yes, my arms and legs started shaking after I fell down.

Past Medical History

- Question
  - Have you had this problem or anything similar before?
  - Do you have any medical problems?
  - Have you been hospitalized before?
  - Have you had any surgeries before?
  - Are you taking any medications?
- Answer
  - No. it's first event.
  - Well, I had some burning during urination. I took antibiotics for one week. This was 5 month ago.

Social History

- Question
  - Do you smoke?
  - How many packs a day?
  - How long have you smoked?
  - Do you drink alcohol?
  - What do you drink?
  - How much do you drink per week?
  - Do you have a lot of stressful situations on your job?
  - Are you exposed to environmental hazard on your job?
- Answer
  - No, I stopped a year ago, I had smoked one pack a day for 25 years.
  - Two to three beers a month.

Family History

- Question
  - Has anyone in your family ever Loss of consciousness like this before?
- Answer
  - Well. My father died from a heart attack at age 53, and my mother died in good health.
  - My father died from lung cancer.

Dialogue

D: Let me introduce myself. My name is Dr. Choi. I'm a doctor working on this hospital. I'm going to ask you some questions and do a physical exam on you. After that I'll discuss with you what I think so far. If you have any questions, I'd be happy to answer them anytime. What made you come to the hospital?

P: I had a blackout this morning.

D: In what situation did you lose your consciousness?

P: I was in school. I didn't feel well, so I stood up to go to the nurse and then fell down.

D: How long did you faint?

P: My friends told me that I woke up soon, just after I fell down.

D: What did you feel before you blacked out?

P: It's hard to describe, but I felt light-headed and nervous.

D: Before you lost your mind, did you have any pain, like a chest pain or headache?

P: No, there was no pain.

D: Did you feel your heart beat fast, or had a hard time breathing?

P: No, there were no other symptoms.

D: Did your body shake after you fell down?

P: No, I just fell down and woke up soon after.

D: Were there any symptoms when you woke up?

P: I couldn't stand right after I woke up, but soon got my strength back.

D: Do you feel dizzy when you stand up?

P: No, it's ok.

D: Do you use a cardiac pace-maker?

P: I don't know what that is.

D: Did this happen to you before?

P: I had a similar experience when I was a elementary school student.

D: Do you have any chronic diseases like diabetes or hypertension?

P: No, I don't.

D: Do you have any heart problems such as arrhythmia?

P: No, my heart is good in shape.

D: Have you got a head trauma before?

P: No, I haven't.

D: Do you take any medications?

P: No.

D: Do you smoke? How much alcohol do you drink?

P: I don't drink or smoke.

D: Do you know any relatives who have similar symptoms?

P: Not that I know of.

3. Chest Pain

Differential Diagnosis

System	Diagnosis
Cardiologic system	MI, angina, pericarditis
Respiratory system	Pulmonary embolism, pnuemonia, pneumothorax
Digestive system	GERD, peptic ulcer disease, esophagitis, esophageal spasm, esophageal rupture, pancreatitis
Musculoskeletal system	Costochondiritis, muscle strain
Aorta	Aortic dissection
Psychiatric	Panic disorder

Onset

발생 시점, 기간에 대해 물어본다.

- Question
  - When did it start?
  - Did it start gradually or abrubtly?
- Answer
  - It started about 1 hour ago while I was working at my desk.
  - It started maybe a year ago.

Location and Radiation

위치, 방사통의 여부에 대해 물어본다.

- Question
  - Where is the exact location of the chest pain?
  - Where do you feel the pain?
  - Does the pain radiate anywhere?
- Answer
  - It hurts in the middle of my chest.
  - It goes to my left arm and neck.

Duration and Frequency

증상이 지속되는 시간과 빈도를 물어본다.

- Question
  - How long have you had this pain?
  - How long does it last at each pain episode?
  - How often do you have a pain?
- Answer
  - It lasts 15 minutes.
  - Maybe three episodes per week.

Quality

통증의 성질(Cardiogenic, Musculoskeletal, Pleuritic, GI)을 물어본다.
양상(짓누르듯이, 조이듯이, 찌르듯이, 쓰리게, 콕콕 쑤시는 느낌), 정도를 물어본다.

- Question
  - Can you describe the pain for me?
  - Is it sharp, dull, burning? Pulsating, cramping, or pressure-like?
  - What is the pain like?
- Answer
  - It is very sharp and worse if I move around.
  - It almost feels like indigestion.
  - It feels like pressure.

Severity

통증의 정도를 물어본다.

- Question
  - On a scale of 1 to 10, with 10 being the worst pain of your life, how would you rate your pain?
  - How much have you had the pain?
  - Did you have a fear of dying or sense of terror with the chest pain?
- Answer
  - On a scale of 1 to 10 where 10 if the worst, this is 7.
  - Yes, I supposed that I could die. That's why I call 911 when it happens.

Context

통증이 발생하는 상황에 대해 물어본다.

- Question
  - What did you do just before the pain started?
  - What did precipitate the chest pain?
- Answer
  - It's unpredictable. I may be in the movies, eating dinner, or driving the car. It can happen anytime.
  - Exertional and postprandial and positional and trauma.

Aggravating and Alleviating Factor

악화와 완화 요인(운동 관련, 자세 관련, 음주, 흡연, 과식, 수면)에 대해 물어본다.

- Question
  - Does anything make the pain better?
  - Does anything make the pain worse?
- Answer
  - Walking makes it worse.
  - Antacids work on this pain.
  - Nothing really.
  - I just try to relax, breathe slow, and it goes away on it's own.

Associated Symptoms

관련 증상(어지러움증, 발열, 호흡곤란, 기침, 객담, 실신, 오심, 구토 등)을 물어본다.

- Question
  - Do you feel nauseated or vomit?
  - Do you have any other symptoms like shortness of breath, palpitations, and dizziness?
- Answer
  - I do feel nauseated right now.
  - I feel nauseated, but I didn't vomit.
  - Yes, I have shortness of breath.
  - No, none of that.

Past Medical History

과거력(관상동맥 중재시술의 여부, 허혈성 심질환, 부정맥, 고혈압, 당뇨)을 물어본다. 특히 cardiac risk factor인 hypertension, hyperlipidemia에 대한 과거력을 물어본다. 약물 복용력에 대해 물어본다.

- Question
  - Do you have any other medical problems?
  - Are you taking any medications for hypertension, diabetes or dyslipidemia?
  - Have you gad any other major illnesses before which include cardiac ischemia or arrhythmia?
  - Have you had any surgeries before?
  - Have you been hospitalized before? If you have, why?

- Answer
  - Never ill before. I have not seen a doctor in 10 years.
  - I have taken hypertension medication for 5 years, treated with a diuretic.
  - I managed the high cholesterol with diet.

Familial History

가족력을 물어본다. 특히 cardiac risk factor로서 familial history of early MI를 확인한다.

- Question
  - Does anyone in your family gave the same problem or anything similar?
  - What did your mother and father die of?
  - Are your family members in good health?
  - Did anyone in your family suffer from early MI?
- Answer
  - My father died of lung cancer at age 72.
  - My mother is alive and has a peptic ulcer.
  - There were no early heart attacks.
  - My brother and father died of heart attacks before the age of 60.

Social History

사회력(직업, 음주, 흡연), 식습관, 외상력에 대해서 물어본다. Cardiac risk factor로서 smoking에 대해 반드시 물어본다.

- Question
  - Do you smoke?
  - How long have you smoked?

- How much alcohol do you drink per week?
- Do you have a lot of stressful situations on your job?
- Did you eat anything unusual lately?
- Has there been any change in your eating habits?

• Answer

- I've smoked two packs per day for 15 years.
- I worked as a stockbroker on Wall Street. It is a stressful job.
- I eat junk food.

Dialogue

D: Let me introduce myself. My name is Dr. Kim. I'm a doctor working on this hospital. I'm going to ask you some questions and do a physical exam on you. After that I'll discuss with you what I think so far. If you have any questions, I'd be happy to answer them anytime. What made you come to this today?

P: I had a chest pain.

D: How long did the pain go?

P: The pain lasted about 5 minutes.

D: Can you point where the pain was most severe?

P: The middle of the chest was most painful.

D: Can you describe how the pain was like?

P: My chest felt tight. It felt like somebody was squeezing my chest.

D: What were you doing when the pain began?

P: I was jogging in a park.

D: Does the pain move, or radiate?

P: The pain radiated to my left arm.

D: On a scale of 1 to 10, saying that 10 is your worst pain in your life, how painful was it?

P: It was about 7 or 8.

D: When does the pain get worse, or better?

P: The pain got better when I stopped running and rested.

D: Do you feel pain when you eat or drink?

P: No, I don't think the pain is related with eating.

D: Are there any other symptoms beside the pain?

P: It was hard to breathe. And I felt dizzy.

D: Do you cough?

P: No, I don't.

D: Is it painful to deeply breathe?

P: No, It's ok.

D: Did these symptoms happen to you before?

P: It happened sometimes, but it wasn't as severe as this time.

D: Do you have any chronic diseases like diabetes or hypertension?

P: I was diagnosed with hypertension 3 years ago.

D: Do you take any medications?

P: I take a anti-hypertensive pill and a pill to lower my cholesterol.

D: Do you smoke?

P: I smoke half-a-pack a day.

D: How long have you smoked cigarette?

P: I smoked for 45 years.

D: How much alcohol do you drink?

P: I drink twice a week.

D: How much do you drink when you do?

P: About a bottle or two.

D: Did you get any surgery recently?

P: I never had a surgery.

D: How much exercise do you do?

P: I started jogging recently.

D: Does any of your relatives have heart disease?

P: My father died of heart attack.

4. Abdominal Pain

Differential Diagnosis

Location	Diagnosis
Hepatobiliary	Hepatitis, choledocholithiasis, cholecystitis, cholangitis, hepatoma
Pancreas, spleen	Pancreatitis, splenic infarct or abscess
Bowel	Gastroduodenitis, peptic ulcer, GERD, appendicitis, diverticulitis, gastroenteritis, ischemic bowel, IBS
Genitourinary system	Nephrolithiasis(renal, ureteral, urethral), ectopic pregnancy, PID, inguinal hernia
Aorta	Acute aortic syndrome(aortic dissection), AAA
기타	Metabolic(DKA, porphyria etc)

Location

증상이 일어나는 위치를 물어본다.

- Question
  - Where do you feel the pain?
  - Can you show me exactly where it is?
- Answer
  - It hurts in the middle of my abdomen.
  - It hurts in the lower part of my abdomen.
  - It's on the right side under my ribs.
  - No special area. It's all over my abdomen.

Onset

증상이 시작된 시간을 물어본다.

- Question
  - When did it start?
  - Did it start gradually or abruptly?
- Answer
  - This has been going on nonstop for 2 days.
  - It has been about 2 months.

Duration and Frequency

증상이 지속되는 시간과 주기성을 물어본다.

- Question
  - How long have you had this pain?
  - How long does it last?
  - Is it constant, or does it come and go?
  - If it comes and goes, how often have you had it?
- Answer
  - Mostly, it's there all the time.
  - It lasts maybe 1 minute, then easy off, like a contraction in labor.

Quality

증상의 양상을 물어본다.

- Question
  - What is the pain like?
  - Can you describe it for me?
  - Is it sharp, dull, burning, pulsating, cramping, or pressure-like?
- Answer
  - It's sharp, like a knife going through me.
  - It's burning and gnawing in nature.
  - It fells like a big crampy pain.

Severity

증상의 강도를 물어본다.

- Question
  - On a scale of 1 to 10, with 10 being the worst pain of your life, how would you rate your pain?
  - How much have you had the pain?
  - Have you ever waken up because of this pain?
- Answer
  - On a scale of 1 to 10, when 10 is the worst, it is 10.

Precipitating Factor

증상의 유발 원인을 물어본다.

- Question
  - What brings the pain on?
  - Do you know what causes the pain to start?
  - Did you eat something in particular recently, like high fat diet, uncooked food or seafood?

Review of Abdominal System

- Question
  - Nausea

    Do you feel nauseated?

    Do you feel sick to your stomach?
  - Vomiting

    Did you vomit?

    Did you throw up?

    What color was the vomit?

    Did you see any blood in it?
- Answer
  - I cannot stop vomiting.
  - I vomited once and I still feel nauseated.
  - I vomited 8 times since last night.

Aggravating and Alleviating Factor

증상의 완화와 악화 인자를 물어본다.

- Question
  - Does anything make the pain better?
  - Does anything make the pain worse?
  - Does the pain get better when you are lying on your side and front and back?
  - Does the pain get better and worse after eating something?
- Answer
  - Lying on my side helps a little.
  - Anything I try to eat or drink will worsen the pain.
  - Lying flat makes pain worse.
  - Alcohol, caffeine, smoking, stress, and not eating make it worse.

Bowel Symptoms

- Question
  - Has there been any change in your bowel movement?
  - Do you have diarrhea? Are you constipated?
  - How long have you had diarrhea and constipation?
  - How many bowel movements do you have per day and week?
  - What does your stool look like?
  - What color is your stool?
  - Is there any mucus or blood in it?
  - Do you feel any pain when you have a bowel movement?
  - Did you travel recently?
- Answer
  - No diarrhea or constipation.

- My last bowel movement was last night and it was brown.
- I have not had a bowel movement for 2 days.

Menstrual History

여성일 경우 월경력에 대해 물어본다.

- Question
  - When was the first day of your last menstrual period?
  - How often do you get your menstrual period?

Past Medical History

과거력을 물어본다.

- Question
  - Have you had similar pain before?
  - Have you had this problem or anything similar before?
  - Do you have any medical problems?
  - Have you been hospitalized before?
  - Have you had any surgeries before?
  - Are you taking any medications?
- Answer
  - I had an attack of pancreatitis from drinking 2 years ago.
  - I had an appendectomy at the age of 22.

Social History

- Question
  - Do you smoke?
  - How many packs a day?
  - How long have you smoked?
  - Do you drink alcohol?
  - What do you drink?
  - How much do you drink per week?
  - Do you have a lot of stressful situations on your job?
  - Are you exposed to environmental hazard on your job?
- Answer
  - I smoke a pack per day.
  - I drink just a beer on Sundays.

Familial History

- Question
  - Does anyone in your family have the same problem or anything similar?
  - What did your mother and father die of?
  - Are your family members in good health?

Dialogue

D: Good morning, Mr. Kim?

P: Good morning.

D: Let me introduce myself. My name is Dr. Lee. I'm a doctor working on this hospital. I'm going to ask you some questions and do a physical exam on you. After that I'll discuss with you what I think so far. If you have any questions, I'd be happy to answer them anytime. What caused you to come in here today?

P: I have a stomachache.

D: Can you show me exactly where it is?

P: It hurts in the upper part of my abdomen.

D: When did it start?

P: Yesterday night.

D: Is it constant, or does it come and go?

P: It's constant.

D: What is the pain like?

P: It's sharp, like a knife going through me.

D: On a scale of 1 to 10, with 10 being the worst pain of your life, how would you rate your pain?

P: It is 10.

D: Do you know what causes the pain to start?

P: I had drunk too much for a number of days.

D: Does anything make the pain worse?

P: Lying on my back makes pain worse.

D: Does anything make the pain better?

P: Stoop myself makes pain better.

D: Do you feel nauseated?

P: No. I don't.

D: Did you vomit?

P: No. I didn't.

D: Do you have diarrhea or constipation?

P: No. I don't.

D: Have you had this problem or anything similar before?

P: No. I haven't.

D: Are you taking any medications?

P: No.

D: Do you smoke?

P: Yes. I do.

D: How many packs a day? And, how long have you smoked?

P: I have smoked a pack per day for 20 years.

D: Do you drink alcohol?

P: Yes. I do.

D: How much do you drink per week?

P: I drink daily 2 pack of soju.

D: Do you have any medical problems?

P: No. I don't

D: Have you had any surgeries before?

P: I had an appendectomy at the age of 22.

D: Does anyone in your family have the same problem or anything similar?

P: No.

5. Dysphagia

Differential Diagnosis

Solid food dysphagia(mechanical problem)	
Intermittent	Lower esophagus(Schatzkis ring)
Progressive	Stricture(has heartburn) Cancer
Solid of liquid dysphagia(neuromuscular problem)	
Intermittent	Diffuse esophageal spasm(has chest pain)
Progressive	Scleroderma(has heartburn) Achalasia(may have respiratory symptoms)

Onset

- Question
  - Do you have a feeling of food sticking in the chest?
  - When did it start?
- Answer
  - Yes, that describes what I'm feeling.
  - It started about 2 months ago.

Nature

- Question
  - What foods do you have problem with swallowing, solid, liquid or both?
  - Do you have pain with swallowing?

- Answer
  - I definitely can't swallow anything solid.
  - Not in the beginning, but now it's getting to the point where swallowing water is becoming a problem.
  - No, I don't have pain.
  - Yes, I do have pain.

Associated Symptoms

- Question
  - Did your weight change recently?
  - Do you have any respiratory symptom, including cough, hoarseness or choking?
- Answer
  - Yes, I've lost 20 pounds in the last month.
  - No, I don't have any cough, hoarseness or choking.

Past History

- Question
  - Did you have any gastrointestinal problems, like gastric reflux or something else?
  - Have you ever had lye ingestion?
- Answer
  - No, I didn't have.
  - No, I have not.

Social History

- Question
  - Do you drink alcohol?
  - What do you drink?
  - How much do you drink per week?
  - Do you smoke?
  - How long have you smoked?
  - How many packs a day?
- Answer
  - I drink just a beer on Sundays.
  - I smoke a pack per day.

Dialogue

D: Good morning, Mr. Kim?

P: Good morning.

D: Let me introduce myself. My name is Dr. Lee. I'm a doctor working on this hospital. I'm going to ask you some questions and do a physical exam on you. After that I'll discuss with you what I think so far. If you have any questions, I'd be happy to answer them anytime. How can I help you?

P: I feel difficult to swallow foods.

D: Do you have a feeling of food sticking in the chest?

P: Yes, that describes what I'm feeling.

D: When did it start?

P: It started about 1 month ago.

D: What foods do you have problem with swallowing, solid, liquid or both?

P: I can't shallow both.

D: Do you have pain with swallowing?

P: Yes, I do have pain.

D: Did your weight change recently?

P: Yes, I've lost 20 pounds in the last month.

D: Do you have any respiratory symptom, including cough, hoarseness or choking?

P: Yes, I have cough.

D: Did you have any gastrointestinal problems, like gastric reflux or something else?

P: No, I didn't have.

D: Have you ever had lye ingestion?

P: No, I have not.

D: Are you taking any medications?

P: No.

D: Do you smoke?

P: No, I don't.

D: Do you drink alcohol?

P: Yes, I do.

D: How much do you drink per week?

P: I drink just a beer per week.

D: Do you have any medical problems?

P: No, I don't.

D: Have you had any surgeries before?

P: No, I have not.

D: Does anyone in your family have the same problem or anything similar?

P: No.

6. Joint and Limb Pain

Differential Diagnosis

1. Trauma
2. Carpal tunnel syndrome
3. Systemic lupus erythematosus
4. Rheumatoid arthritis
5. Psoriatic arthritis
6. Fracture
7. Osteoarthritis
8. Stress fracture
9. Peripheral vascular disease

Key history

- *Location, quality, intensity, duration, pattern, associated symptoms, exacerbating and alleviating factors, trauma, medications, DVT risk factors, alcohol and drug use, family history of rheumatic disease*

Onset and Duration

나타나는 통증에 대해 물어본다.

- Question
  - When did the pain first start?
  - How often does it hurt during the day?
  - How long does the pain go?
  - Does it hurt at a particular time of day?
- Answer
  - About 2 days ago.
  - About 5 times a day.
  - About 2~3 hours.
  - It usually hurts in the morning.

Character and Alleviating, Aggravating Factor

- Question
  - Has the pain gone worse than before?
  - What is the pain like?
  - Is there anything that alleviates the pain?
  - Is there anything that makes the pain worse?
- Answer
  - Yes, it aches more than before.
  - It's like as if something is biting over it.
  - Putting an icepack over it makes it better.
  - It hurts a lot after I work out.

Associated Joint Symptoms

관절 부위에 다른 증상이 있는지 물어본다.

- Question
  - Is there any swelling at the pain site?
  - Is there any trouble moving your joints at the pain site?
  - Is there any numbness around?
- Answer
  - My knees are swollen a lot.
  - My fingers are very stiff.
  - I can't feel anything below my knees.

Accompanying Symptoms

동반되는 관절 외 증상이 있는지 물어본다.

• Question

- Are there any muscle cramps?
- Do you think you feel any pain in the bones?
- Do you have any problems swallowing?
- You don't have any trouble breathing?

• Answer

- I think I have a back muscle pain.
- I'm not sure which it hurts.
- Yes, it's hard to eat my food.
- No, I don't see any problem.

Social, Familial History

사회력, 가족력에 대해 물어본다.

• Question

- What do you do for a living?
- Do you exercise regularly?
- Do you have anyone in your family with the same symptoms?

• Answer

- I work at a construction site, moving heavy machinery.
- I go to the gym everyday.
- My brother has a shoulder pain on the left.

7. Low Back Pain

Differential Diagnosis

1. Disk herniation
2. Lumbar muscle strain
3. Lumbar spinal stenosis
4. Kidney stone
5. Pyelonephritis
6. Arthritis

Key history

- *Location, quality, intensity, radiation, context, associated symptoms, exacerbating and alleviating factors, history of cancer, recurrent UTIs, diabetes, renal stones, IV drug use*

Location and Time and Character

통증이 나타나는 위치, 기간, 양상에 대해 물어본다.

• Question

- Where is the exact location of the pain?
- Since when did it start to hurt?
- What is the pain like?
- How often does it hurt?

• Answer

- It is in the middle of my lower back.
- It started yesterday. I took 2 tylenols but it didn't help.
- It is like a dull throbbing pain.
- It is continuous.

Past Medical History

과거력에 대해 물어본다.

- Question
  - Do you have any underlying disease?
  - Have you hurt your back in the past?
  - Are you taking any drugs?
  - Do you have anyone in your family with rheumatoid arthritis?
- Answer
  - I have lung cancer.
  - I fell down on the stairs 2 years ago.
  - I'm taking steroids.
  - My mother was diagnosed with it.

Dialogue

D: Good morning, Mr. Kim?

P: Good morning.

D: Let me introduce myself. My name is Dr. Lee. I'm a doctor working on this hospital. I'm going to ask you some questions and do a physical exam on you. After that I'll discuss with you what I think so far. If you have any questions, I'd be happy to answer them anytime. What caused you to come in here today?

P: I have a joint pain.

D: When did the pain first start?

P: About 2 weeks ago.

D: How often does it hurt during the day?

P: About 5 times a day.

D: How long does the pain go?

P: About 2~3 hours.

D: Does it hurt at a particular time of day?

P: It usually hurts in the morning.

D: Has the pain gone worse than before?

P: Yes, it aches more than before.

D: Is there any swelling at the pain site?

P: Yes, my knees are swollen a lot.

D: Have you been hurt in your joints or over used it?

P: No.

D: Do you have difficulty moving your joint over than 1 hour in the morning?

P: Yes, It keeps on about 1 hour and than it gets better.

D: Is the pain in your joints symmetric?

P: Yes.

D: Did your weight change recently?

P: Yes, I've lost 10 pounds in the last month.

D: Are you taking any medications?

P: No.

D: Do you smoke?

P: No.

D: Do you drink alcohol?

P: No.

D: Do you have any medical problems?

P: No.

D: Have you had any surgeries before?

P: No.

D: Does anyone in your family gave the same problem or anything similar?

P: No.

D: What do you do for a living?

P: I'm a teacher.

8. Dizziness

Differential Diagnosis

Meniere's disease	Usually lasing 1~8 hours and low-frequency hearing loss
Orthostatic hypotension due to dehydration	Diarrhea and loop diuretic use Melena(GI bleeding)
Benign paroxysmal positional vertigo (BPPV)	Transient vertigo following changes in head position but not associated with hearing loss
Labyrinthitis	This frequently follows a viral infection (usually URI) and is accompanied by hearing loss and tinnitus. Vertigo is usually continuous lasts several days to a week.
Acoustic neuroma	More commonly causes continuous dysequilibrium rather than episodic vertigo.

Onset

- Question
  - When did it start?
  - Is dizziness always there or does it come and go?
- Answer
  - It started 2 days ago.
  - Come and go.

Progression and Duration

- Question
  - Is it getting worse?
  - How long does it last?
  - How long have you had this dizziness?
- Answer
  - It is getting worse.
  - It last for 20~30 minutes.
  - It can happen anytime.

Quality

- Question
  - Can you describe the meaning of dizziness?
  - Tell me exactly what you mean by dizziness.
  - Did you feel the room spinning around you, or did you feel lightheaded as if you were going to pass out?
  - Did you black out?
- Answer
  - Well, I feel as if the room were spinning around me.

Precipitating Factor

- Question
  - What causes this dizziness to happen?

Aggravating and Alleviating Factor

- Question
  - Does anything make the dizziness worse?
  - Tell me about positions that can elicit the dizziness. for example lying down, sitting, standing up.
  - What makes you feel better?
- Answer
  - Closing my eyes and staying very still help.
  - When I get up from bed or lie down to sleep, but as I said, it can happen anytime.

Associated Symptoms

- Question
  - Have you noticed anything else besides your dizziness?
  - Did you notice any change in your hearing?
  - Do your ears ring?
  - Do you feel nauseated?
  - Do you vomit?
  - Do you have any recent infection?
  - Did you lose consciousness?
- Answer
  - Yes, I have difficulty hearing you in my left ear. This started yesterday.
  - I feel nauseated, and vomited several times.
  - I have had really bad diarrhea. I've had it for the past 3 days, but it is much better today.

Past Medical History

- Question
  - Have you had this problem or anything similar before?
  - Have you had any accidents or injuries before?
  - Do you have any medical problems?
  - Have you been hospitalized before?
  - Have you had any surgeries before?
  - Are you taking any medications?
  - Are you taking any over-the-counter drugs, vitamins, or herb?
- Answer
  - High blood pressure, diagnosed 7 years ago.
  - Furosemide, and captopril.

Social History

- Question
  - Do you smoke?
  - How many packs a day?
  - How long have you smoked?
  - Do you drink alcohol?
  - What do you drink?
  - How much do you drink per week?
  - Do you have a lot of stressful situations on your job?
  - Are you exposed to environmental hazard on your job?
- Answer
  - No. I'm not a smoker.
  - I drink 2~3 beers a week.

Dialogue

D: Good morning, Ms. Lee?

P: Good morning.

D: Let me introduce myself. My name is Dr. Kim. I'm a doctor working on this hospital. I'm going to ask you some questions and do a physical exam on you. After that I'll discuss with you what I think so far.

P: OK.

D: If you have any questions, I'd be happy to answer them anytime. How can I help you today? What brought you here today?

P: I came here for my dizziness.

D: Did you feel the room spinning around you, or did you feel lightheaded as if you were going to pass out?

P: I felt as if the room were spinning around me.

D: OK. When did it start?

P: Today in the morning.

D: Do you have dizziness now?

P: No. I'm OK now.

D: Then when you have it, how long does it last?

P: About 30 seconds I think.

D: Can you tell me the situation around your dizziness?

P: After waking up in this morning, I tried to sit on my bed. At that time I suddenly felt it.

D: Have it occurred after that time?

P: Yes. It can happen anytime I move my head.

D: Do you have any other symptom with dizziness?

P: Nothing special I think.

D: I'll ask you some symptoms you might have had. Did you notice any change in your hearing?

P: No, I don't.

D: Do your ears ring?

P: No.

D: Do you feel nauseated?

P: No.

D: Do you vomit?

P: No.

D: Did you lose consciousness?

P: No, I don't.

D: Have you had accidents or injury on your head before?

P: No, I have not.

D: Do you have any recent infection?

P: No, I don't.

D: Have you ever had similar symptoms before?

P: No, this morning was the first time.

D: Do you have any medical problems?

P: No.

D: Have you been hospitalized before?

P: No.

D: Have you had any surgeries before?

P: No.

D: Are you taking any medications?

P: No.

D: Are you taking any over-the-counter drugs, vitamins, or herb?

P: No.

D: Do you smoke?

P: No.

D: Do you drink alcohol?

P: Yes.

D: How much do you drink per week?

P: I drink 2~3 beers a week.

D: Do you have any family member who had brain disease?

P: No.

9. Confusion and Memory Loss

Differential Diagnosis

Alzheimer's disease	Insidious onset, with steady, progress decline in cognitive function over years
Vascular (multi-infarct) dementia	Given the patient's history of atherosclerotic vascular disease (stroke, MI)
Depression with pseudodementia	More noticeable after death of the patient's family
Hypothyroidism	Edema, weight gain
Vitamin B12 deficiency	A prior bowel resection
Subdural hematoma	Given the patient's history of falls and head trauma

Onset

- Question
  - When did it start?
- Answer
  - I can't remember exactly, but my daughter told me that I started forgetting last year.

Progression

- Question
  - Is it getting worse?
- Answer
  - My daughter has told me that it is getting worse.

Severity

- Question
  - What are things that are difficult to remember?
- Answer
  - Turning off the stove, my phone number, my keys, the way to my home, the names of my friends.

Daily Activity

- Question
  - Do you need any help getting dressed?
  - What do you need help with when you eat?
  - Can you tell me about your (shopping, cooking, money management, housework, telephone use, and travel outside the home)?
- Answer
  - I have some trouble with these, and I need help sometimes.
  - I did take the wrong bus a few times.
  - My house is a mess.
  - I did forget to pay my rent 3 months in a row, but that's normal for people my age, isn't it?

Associated Symptoms

- Question
  - Urinary incontinence

    Has there been any change in your urinary habits?

    Do you feel as though you have very little time to make it to the bathroom once you feel the urge to urinate?

- Feeling (sad, depressed)

  Do you feel guilty about anything?

  How is your energy level?

  What interest or pleasure in your daily activities?
- Difficulty sleeping

  Do you have any problems falling asleep?

  How many hours do you sleep?
- Weight

  Have you noticed any change in your weight?
- Head trauma

  Have you had any accidents or injuries before?
- Visual change

  Do you notice any change in your vision?
- Weakness and numbness and paresthesia

  Do you notice any numbness or weakness?
- Speech difficulties

  Do you notice any speech difficulties?
- Do you have any light-headedness or feeling faint?

• Answer
- I think so. I had a large bruise on the side of my head a while back.
- Yes, I have weakness in my left arm from a stroke I had a long time ago.
- I feel upset because of all of this.
- Only if I stand up too quickly, I feel faint.

Past Medical History

• Question
- Have you had any accidents or injuries before?
- Do you have any medical problems?
- Have you been hospitalized before?

- Have you had any surgeries before?
- Are you taking any medications?

• Answer

- I have high blood pressure, for a long time.
- I don't know medications names.
- I had a bowel obstruction a long time ago, and they removed part of my intestine.

Social History

• Question

- Do you smoke?
- How many packs a day?
- How long have you smoked?
- Do you drink alcohol?
- What do you drink?
- How much do you drink per week?
- Do you have a lot of stressful situations on your job?
- Are you exposed to environmental hazard on your job?

• Answer

- I smoke a pack per day.
- I drink just a beer on Sundays.

Family History

응급 상황에 도움이 있는지 물어본다.

• Question

- Has anyone in your family had ever confusion and memory loss like this?
- Who support your daily activity?

- Answer
  - No.
  - I live with my daughter.

Dialogue

D: Good morning, Ms. Lee?

P: Good morning.

D: Let me introduce myself. My name is Dr. Kim. I'm a doctor working on this hospital. I'm going to ask you some questions and do a physical exam on you. After that I'll discuss with you what I think so far.

P: OK.

D: If you have any questions, I'd be happy to answer them anytime. How can I help you today? What brought you here today?

P: I can't remember things easily.

D: When did it start?

P: I can't remember exactly, but my daughter told me that I started forgetting last year.

D: Is it getting worse?

P: I think it is getting worse.

D: What are things that are difficult to remember?

P: Turning off the stove, my phone number, my keys.

D: Do you need any help getting dressed?

P: No. I can do it myself.

D: Do you need help when you eat?

P: No. I can do it myself.

D: Can you tell me about your housework?

P: It's going well, except I sometimes forget to turn off the stove.

D: Has there been any change in your urinary habits?

P: Yes. I sometimes urinate when I cough or laugh.

D: Do you feel guilty about anything?

P: Not actually.

D: Do you have any problems falling asleep?

P: Well. I sleep about 5 hours a day, but I think that's enough.

D: Do you feel depressed?

P: No.

D: Have you noticed any change in your weight?

P: No, I have not.

D: Do you notice any change in your vision?

P: No, I don't

D: Do you notice any numbness or weakness?

P: Yes, but I think that's because I'm old.

D: Do you feel difficulty to move your body recently?

P: Not actually.

D: Do you notice any speech difficulties?

P: Well. Sometimes I can't remember some words. But I can communicate well.

D: Have you had any accidents or injuries before?

P: I broke my arm by car accident when I was 6 years old.

D: Do you have any medical problems?

P: I have been diagnosed for hypertension 5 years ago.

D: Have you ever heard that you have high blood cholesterol level before?

P: Yes, I have.

D: Have you been hospitalized before?

P: No.

D: Have you had any surgeries before?

P: No.

D: Are you taking any medications?

P: Yes, I take hypertension drugs.

D: Do you know about the drug?

P: No, I don't.

D: Do you smoke?

P: No, I don't.

D: Do you drink alcohol?

P: Yes, I do.

D: How much do you drink per week?

P: I drink just a bottle of beer on Sundays.

D: Has anyone in your family had ever memory loss like this?

P: I don't know.

D: Who support your daily activity?

P: I live with my daughter.

D: Alright. I'll ask you some question to test your memory and concentration power. Some may be easy but some may be hard. Don't be too nervous. What's the day today?

P: It's Friday.

D: What's the date today?

P: It's 2011 June 3rd.

D: What season is it?

P: It's Summer.

D: Can you tell me what city are you in?

P: Seoul.

D: What is this place for?

P: To treat patients.

D: I will test your memory. Please remember these words. I'll ask you later. Airplane, Pine tree, Pencil. Can you tell me what they are?

P: Airplane, Pine tree, Pencil.

D: What is this?

P: It's a watch.

D: Then, What's this?

P: It's a computer.

D: OK. Please turn this paper upside down and fold it by half and then give it to me. Please listen and repeat after me. One picture is worth a thousand words.

P: One picture is worth a thousand words.

D: OK. Please draw this figure in this paper. Can you remember 3 words I told you a few minutes ago?

P: They were Airplane, Pine tree, Pencil.

10. Cough and Shortness of Breath

Differential Diagnosis

〈Cough〉

System		Diagnosis
Respiratory system	Acute cough	URI, acute sinusitis, allergic rhinitis, COPD acute exacerbation, pertussis
	Subacute cough	Acute, chronic sinusitis, postinfectious cough, asthma, pertussis
	Chronic cough	Postnasal drip, asthma, chronic bronchitis, COPD, bronchiectasis, lung cancer
Other systems		GERD. Side effect of ACE inhibitor, psychogenic cough, left heart failure, mass(thymoma)

〈Shortness of breath〉

System	Diagnosis
Respiratory system	Asthma, bronchitis, pneumonitis, pneumonia, COPD, bronchiectasis, lung cancer, lung abscess, tuberculosis, pulmonary fibrosis, sarcoidosis, pulmonary embolus
Cardiologic system	CHF, cardiac valvular disease, pericarditis
Gastrointestinal system	GERD
Others	Foreign body, psychogenic, anemia, pneumothorax, hemothorax

Onset

기침과 호흡곤란의 시작에 대해 물어본다. 특히 기침과 같은 증상들은 그것이 시작된 시점에 따라 3주 이내는 Acute, 3주 이상은 Chronic, 3~8주는 Subacute라 한다.

- Question
  - When did it start?
  - How long have you had the cough and shortness of breath?
  - Was the onset of shortness of breath sudden or gradual?
- Answer
  - It started 2 hours ago.

Precipitating Factor

증상의 유발 원인에 대해 물어본다.

- Question
  - Tell me what happens before your cough.
  - What causes the cough to start?
  - When do you feel short of breath?
  - What were you doing at the time the shortness of breath started?
- Answer
  - There is nothing special which makes me start to cough. I cough all the time.
  - I were running in gym class.

Quality

기침의 양상, 증상이 계속해서 악화되는지 여부를 물어본다.

- Question
  - Are there any changes of the cough during the day?
  - Do you bring up any sputum with your cough, or is it dry?
  - Do you cough at night?
  - Do you wake up in the middle of the night short of breath?
- Answer
  - Yes, the cough is productive of sputum.
  - Especially at night. I sometimes can't sleep because of the annoying cough.
  - It has progressively worsened over the 6 weeks. I couldn't take it anymore, so last night I went to the emergency room.
  - Yes, that was happening to me.

Severity and Quantity

기침의 심한 정도, 호흡곤란이 어느 정도 되는지를 물어본다.

- Question
  - How often do you cough?
  - Do you get short of breath when you're climbing stairs?
  - How many steps can you climb before you get short of breath?
  - How far do you walk on level ground before you have shortness of breath?
- Answer
  - Yes, when I walk up the stairs, I get shortness of breath.

Aggravating and Alleviating Factor

어떤 경우에 기침과 호흡곤란이 완화되고 악화되는지 물어본다. 찬 공기, 운동, 작업장 노출에 대한 병력 청취, 호흡곤란에서는 특히 자세에 의한 악화, 완화에 대한 병력 청취가 필요하다.

- Question
  - Does anything make it better?
  - Does anything make it worse?
  - What makes the shortness of breath worse?
- Answer
  - It gets better when I sit up and prop myself up.
  - It sets worse with exertion and when I lie flat.

Review of Respiratory System

특히 기침 환자에게는 sputum에 대해 물어보는 것이 매우 중요하다.

- Question
  - Presence and description of sputum
    What color is it?
    Is there any blood in it?
  - Can you estimate the amount of the phlegm? A teaspoon? A tablespoon? A cupful?
  - Have you been wheezing?
- Answer
  - There is some brownish sputum. The color was yellowish mucus.
  - I noticed a teaspoon amount of blood yesterday.
  - Yes, I have and haven't.

Associated Symptoms

기침할 때 동반 증상에 대해 물어본다.

• Question
  - Do you have a fever?
  - Do you have chills?
  - Have you noticed any fluid retention around your ankles?
  - Do you have to prop yourself up on pillows in order to sleep at night? How many?

• Answer
  - Yes, I have a fever and chills.
  - Lately, my temperature has been 101°F almost everyday.
  - Yes, my ankles are sometimes swollen.
  - Yes, I have been sleeping on three or four pillows recently. I can't seem to sleep lying flat like in the past.

Past Medical History

만성 질환 여부(당뇨병, 고혈압, 결핵 등)와 약물 복용력(ACE inhibitor 등)을 반드시 물어보고, 기침이나 호흡곤란을 일으킬 수 있는 기저 질환으로서 심장 질환이나 폐 질환의 유무, 류머티스열, 승모판 협착증, 알레르기 질환 등의 과거력을 물어본다.

• Question
  - Have you had any other major illnesses before?
  - Do you have any other medical problems like diabetes, hypertension or Tb?
  - Are you taking any medications?
  - Do you have any allergies?

- Have you been hospitalized before?
- Have you had any surgeries before?

• Answer

- I have high blood pressure for 5 years.
- I have no history of asthma, Tb, or pneumonia.

Familial History

심폐 질환, 출혈성 질환 등에 대해 물어본다.

• Question

- Does anyone in your family have asthma or allergy?
- Are the members in your family in good health? Does anyone have the same problem or anything similar?

Social History

흡연 여부, 직업 등에 대해 물어본다.

• Question

- Do you smoke?
- Have you ever smoked before?
- How many packs a day?
- How long have you smoked?
- What type of work do you do?

• Answer

- I don't smoke.

- I've smoked 10 cigarettes a day for 3 years.
- I've been meaning to stop smoking.
- I work as a cashier in a toy store.

Dialogue

D: Good morning, Ms. Lee?

P: Good morning.

D: Let me introduce myself. My name is Dr. Kim. I'm a doctor working on this hospital. I'm going to ask you some questions and do a physical exam on you. After that I'll discuss with you what I think so far.

P: OK.

D: If you have any questions, I'd be happy to answer them anytime. What brought you here today?

P: I can't breathe well.

D: How long have you had the shortness of breath?

P: About 2 years.

D: Was the onset of shortness of breath sudden or gradual?

P: It is getting worse since it appeared 2 years ago.

D: Did you go to hospital for that reason?

P: No. I thought it would be OK soon.

D: When do you feel short of breath?

P: When exercise.

D: What were you doing at the time the shortness of breath started?

P: I sit down on the ground and rest for some time.

D: Do you wake up in the middle of the night because of short of breath?

P: No, I don't.

D: Do you get short of breath when you're climbing stairs?

P: Yes.

D: How many steps can you climb before you get short of breath?

P: I will have breathing difficulty when I climb 3rd floor by stairs.

D: How far do you walk on level ground before you have shortness of breath?

P: About 500 meters.

D: Do you get breathing difficulty when you are at rest?

P: No.

D: Do you cough?

P: No, I don't.

D: Do you have a fever?

P: No, I don't.

D: Do you have chills?

P: No.

D: Have you noticed any fluid retention around your ankles?

P: Yes, my ankles are sometimes swollen.

D: Have you had any other major illnesses before?

P: What is major illness?

D: Medical problems like Diabetes, hypertension, tuberculosis. Do you have high blood sugar?

P: No, I don't.

D: Do you have high blood pressure?

P: No, I don't.

D: Have you been diagnosed as tubuerculosis?

P: No, I have not.

D: Are you taking any medications?

P: No, I am not.

D: Do you have any allergies?

P: No, I don't.

D: Have you been hospitalized before?

P: No, I have not.

D: Have you had any surgeries before?

P: No.

D: Does anyone in your family have asthma or allergy?

P: No.

D: Does anyone have the same problem or anything similar?

P: No.

D: Do you smoke?

P: I don't smoke.

D: What do you do for earning?

P: I work as a cashier in a grocery store.

11. Hematuria and Other Urinary Symptoms

Differential Diagnosis

Upper urinary tract	- renal cell carcinoma - glomerulonephritis
Lower urinary tract	- bladder cancer - Urolitihiasis - UTI
Others	- BPH - Prostate cancer

Key history

- *Amount, duration, clots, associated symptoms, medications, history of vigorous exercise, trauma, smoking, stones, cancer, or easy bleeding*

Nature

혈뇨의 성질에 대해 물어본다.

- Question
  - What was the color of your urine like?
- Answer
  - It was dark, coca-cola colored.
  - It was a pinkish bloody red color.
  - Normal, I was told that I had hematuria by my general physician on my urine tests.

Onset and Duration

혈뇨의 발생 시기, 지속 시간, 양에 대해 물어본다.

- Question
  - How many time did you see blood when urinating?
  - How much blood do you think was in your urine?
- Answer
  - Once a day, usually at the gym after I work out.
  - Only in the morning, right after I get up.
  - It was bloody from the beginning till the end.
  - It was red only for the first few seconds.

Pain

통증이 동반되는지 물어본다.

- Question
  - Is there any place that hurts?
  - Since when did it start to hurt?
  - What is the quality of the pain?
  - How is the pain progressing?
  - Does the pain stretch to anywhere else?
- Answer
  - Right here, on the left side of the back.
  - It started about 3 hours ago.
  - It is like someone is punching me in the side.
  - It seems to be getting worse. I need pain medications.
  - It seems to be going into my left groin area.

Accompanying Symptoms 1

동반 증상이 있는지 물어본다.

- Question
  - Do you having any problems when urinating?
  - Do you have a fever right now?
  - Have you been loosing some weight recently?
  - Are you having any kind of abdominal pain?
- Answer
  - I feel as if there is some left in my bladder.
  - I have to push some power to urinate.

Factors

혈뇨의 유발 요인에 대해 물어본다.

- Question
  - Have you had any physical injuries recently?
  - Have you been working out hard recently?
  - Are you in your period now?
  - Are you taking any kind of drugs?
- Answer
  - Just some marijuana now and then.
  - My general physician prescribed me with rifampin.

Associated Symptoms

배뇨 습관에 변화가 있는지 물어본다.

- Question
  - Have you felt some changes when urinating?
  - Were there any changes in you urine?
- Answer
  - I don't feel that I've emptied enough.
  - It hurts in my lower stomach when I go to the restroom.
  - I think there was some blood.
  - It's changed very foamy lately.

Severity

일상생활에 얼마나 지장을 주는지 알아본다.

- Question
  - Do you urinate while you're in bed?
  - Did you ever feel that you would not make it to the bathroom on time?
  - Have you ever urinated before reaching the bathroom?
- Answer
  - I have to get up every night about 3 times.
  - It happens 3~4 times a day. It's hard to concentrate on my work.
  - Once, I had to go to home to change.

Onset

발생 시기에 대해 물어본다.

- Question
  - How many times did you have this kind of problem?
  - When did this first happen?
- Answer
  - Almost every time I have to go to the restroom.
  - About 2 years ago. But it has become worse lately.
  - After I had my second baby.

Accompanying Symptoms 2

동반된 증상이 있는지 물어본다.

- Question
  - Are there any other problems you have?
  - Do you have any other symptoms?
- Answer
  - I feel kind of nauseous.
  - I think I have a fever.
  - I think there is some blood in my urine.

Dialogue

D: Good morning, Ms. Lee?

P: Good morning.

D: Let me introduce myself. My name is Dr. Kim. I'm a doctor working on this hospital. I'm going to ask you some questions and do a physical exam on you. After that I'll discuss with you what I think so far.

P: OK.

D: If you have any questions, I'd be happy to answer them anytime. How can I help you today? What brought you here today?

P: I think I'm having a blood in my urine.

D: Ah··· You must be worried. What was the color of your urine?

P: It was red. Just like blood.

D: How much blood was in your urine?

P: The whole urine was red.

D: Was there anything like blood clot in your urine too?

P: No. I don't think so.

D: When did it happen?

P: Today morning. I went to the bathroom after I woke up and it happened. I was totally freaked out and ran down to here right away.

D: Was there any pain when you urinate?

P: Well··· I'm not sure. It wasn't that painful.

D: Was the urine foamy?

P: No, it wasn't.

D: Were there any uncomfortable symptoms when you urinate this morning or before?

P: Nothing special.

D: Are you feeling chilly? Or do you have any fever?

P: Not at all.

D: Did you lose weight recently?

P: No, actually I'm concerned because I'm gaining weight.

D: Is it like swelling?

P: No. It's not like that I just haven't worked out recently.

D: Is there any pain on your flank or back?

P: I had a very severe pain in my right flank 10 minutes after dinner yesterday and then it got better. Also I woke up about at two in the morning because of the pain was relapsed. Few minutes later I was OK and then back to sleep.

D: It must be very painful if you woke up because of that. Have you had serious cold or sore throat recently?

P: Nope.

D: Have you been injured on your flank or abdomen recently?

P: No, I haven't.

D: Do you have gum bleeding? or get bruise a lot?

P: No, not at all.

D: Now I'm going to ask about your past, familial and social history. Have you heard about you having something unusual in your urine tests before?

P: No.

D: Have you had bloody urine after severe exercise?

P: No.

D: Do you have any medical problems?

P: No. I was healthy all the time. So I was more concerned today.

D: Do you take any drug?

P: No.

D: Is there anyone in your family who has bloody urine like you or kidney problem?

P: No. There isn't.

12. Amenorrhea

Differential Diagnosis

Primary amenorrhea	- Turner syndrome - Imperforated hymen
Secondary amenorrhea	- Pregnancy - Polycystic ovary syndrome - Amenorrhea secondary to prolactinoma - Menopause - Sheehan's syndrome - Anorexia nervosa

Key history

- *Primary and secondary, duration, possible pregnancy, associated symptoms, history of anorexia nervosa, excessive dieting, vigorous exercise, DandCs, uterine infections, drug use, medications*

Menstrual History

월경, 기본 산과력에 대해 물어본다.

• Question

- When was your last period?
- How regular are your periods?
- When was your last intercourse?
- When was your first period?

• Answers

- It was about 2 months ago.
- I used to have regular periods every month lasting 4~5 days, but over the last year I started having them less frequently, every 5~6 weeks lasting for seven days.
- It was when I was in 6th grade.

Primary Amenorrhea

1차성 무월경에 대해 물어본다.

• Question
  - Did you go through normal puberty?
  - Was there any kind of pain?
  - Are you known of any genetic diseases?
• Answer
  - Yes, I was a bit earlier than my friends.
  - No, I haven't grown any hair in my pubic areas.
  - Yes, I had a pelvic pain every month, but there wasn't any bleeding.

Secondary Amenorrhea

2차성 무월경에 대해 물어본다.

• Question
  - Are you taking your meals regularly?
  - Did you happen to find any discharges coming out of your breasts?
  - Are you feeling any hot flashes or cold sweats?
• Answer
  - My appetite has been not so good recently.
  - Something white did come out, could it be milk?
  - Yes, my face has been burning up once in a while.

13. Vaginal Bleeding

Differential Diagnosis

1. Dysfunctional uterine bleeding
2. Endometrial cancer
3. Cervical cancer
4. Spontaneous abortion
5. Ectopic pregnancy
6. Pelvic inflammatory disease
7. Atropic vaginitis

Key history

- *Pre-vs. postmenopausal, duration, amount, menstrual history, associated discharge, pelvic or abdominal pain, urinary symptoms, trauma, medications, history of PAP smears*

Bleeding

출혈 양상에 대해 물어본다.

- Question
  - When did this bleeding first start?
  - How many pads were soaked? Was it more or less than your normal menstrual period?
  - Is the bleeding getting worse?
  - What were you doing when you started bleeding?
- Answer
  - It started about 5 hours ago.
  - Just one pad, like the first day of my period, but I'm afraid.
  - I think it is slowing down.

Menstrual History

월경력에 대해 물어보고 비교해 본다.

- Question
  - When was your last menstrual period?
  - Are you having any abdominal pain?
  - Did you have any sexual intercourse recently?
- Answer
  - It was 9 weeks ago.
  - Some cramps, like my period.

14. Vaginal Discharge

Differential Diagnosis

1. Bacterial vaginosis
2. Vaginitis - candidal
3. Vaginitis - trichomonal
4. Cervicitis (chlamydia, gonorrhea)

Key history

- *Amount, color, consistency, odor, duration, associated vaginal burning pain, pruritis, recent sexual activity, onset of last menstrual period, use of contraceptives, tampons, history of sexually transmitted diseases.*

Discharge

질 분비물의 양상에 대해 물어본다.

- Question
  - What color was the discharge?
  - Was there any smell from the discharge?
  - Were there any other symptoms noticeable?
  - Does your partner have any other symptoms?
- Answer
  - It was yellowish white.
  - No, I wasn't able to notice any scent.
  - The area itches a lot.
  - No, there's nothing wrong with my husband.

Dialogue

D: Good morning, Ms. Lee?

P: Good morning.

D: Let me introduce myself. My name is Dr. Kim. I'm a doctor working on this hospital. I'm going to ask you some questions and do a physical exam on you. After that I'll discuss with you what I think so far.

P: OK.

D: If you have any questions, I'd be happy to answer them anytime. How can I help you today? What brought you here today?

P: I'm here because I don't menstruate.

D: Ah··· You must be worried. How long have you been missing your period?

P: About 6 months.

D: When was your first period?

P: When I was 13.

D: You are 19 now.

P: Yes.

D: Are you sexually active?

P: No. I'm not.

D: How is your normal period like?

P: I haven't had normal one month period since my first one. I'm always having it 3 to 6 months and I have a heavy flow everytime.

D: Do you have cramps?

P: No, not really.

D: Is there any weight change recently?

P: Well··· Not recent but I'm gaining weight constantly.

D: Is there change in your diet?

P: No, I eat like usual.

D: Did you have severe exercise recently?

P: Nothing special.

D: Are you in a stressful condition recently?

P: Just a little bit because of my mid-term exam.

D: Do you have changes of your voice tone? or lots of hair growing, or pimples?

P: Yeah. As you can see I have a lot of hair and pimples. Does this have to do something with my symptoms?

D: I can't sure you now, but I think it's related. Are you taking any medicines?

P: No. I don't.

D: Is there any abnormal discharge from your nipples?

P: Nope.

D: Are you feeling any hot flashes or cold sweats?

P: No.

D: Are you feeling very tired or exhausted recently?

P: No.

D: Now I'm going to ask about your past, familial and social history. Do you have any underlying disease?

P: No, not at all.

D: Do you smoke?

P: No.

D: Does your mother or sister has similar symptoms?

P: No.

15. Child with Fever

Differential Diagnosis

아이 없이 부모만 와서 아이의 상태를 설명해 줌.

1. URI
2. UTI
3. Meningitis
4. Gastroenteritis
5. Measles
6. Rubella

Key history

- *Severity, duration, associated localizing symptoms, appetite, rash, sick contacts, day care, immunizations, past history*

Character and Time

발열의 양상, 빈도, 기간

- Question
  - When did the child's temperature begin to rise?
  - How high was it?
  - Was the temperature high the whole time?
- Answer
  - About 2 days ago.
  - I measured it at home and it was 38°C.
  - No, the fever came on and off.

Accompanying Symptoms

동반되는 다른 증상이 있는지 물어본다.

[General]

- Question
  - Does your child have any chills?
- Answer
  - Yes, she's been shaking all day.

[Respiratory]

- Question
  - Does she have some trouble breathing?
  - Is she feeling any pain in her neck?
- Answer
  - Yes, I can see her breathing heavily.
  - Yes, she has some sort of rash on her face and chest.
  - Yes, she says her neck hurts every time she swallows.

[Dermatology]

- Question
  - Are there any noticeable rashes on her body?
  - When did the rash first appear?
- Answer
  - It started 2 days ago on her face and then spread to her chest, back and belly.

[Gastrointestinal]

- Question
  - Was there any vomiting?
  - Have you noticed any changes in her stool?

- How about her bowel habits?

- Answer
  - I think there has been a lot of diarrhea lately.

Life Style

[Urology]

- Question
  - Was there anything unusual in her urine?
- Answer
  - No, there wasn't.
  - There wasn't anything unusual.

[Appetite]

- Question
  - Has she been eating well lately?
- Answer
  - Yes, despite the fever, she is eating really well.

[Sleep]

- Question
  - Does she sleep well at night?
- Answer
  - No, she had to wake up a couple times because of the fever.

Past Medical History

약물 복용에 대해 물어본다.

- Question
  - Has she been treated with antibiotics?
  - Is he being treated with any kind of chemotherapy?
  - Has she taken any medications recently?
- Answer
  - She has taken some Tylenol.
  - Yes, she is being treated for leukemia.
  - Yes, they were prescribed last week when she caught a cold.

과거 병력, 백신접종 여부에 대해 물어본다.

- Question
  - Has she been getting her vaccinations regularly?
  - Does she have a record for any surgery or drug allergies?
  - Has she been ill recently?
- Answer
  - 3 months ago she had an ear infection that was treated successfully with amoxicillin.
  - No, she doesn't.
  - She's been getting them up to date.

Precipitating Factor

아이가 감염의 가능성이 있으므로, 병원균에 노출될 수 있는 감염 경로에 대해 물어본다.

• Question

- Does she go to any daycare centers?
- Were there any other children there who had the same symptoms as her?
- Is there anyone in the family who has been ill recently?

• Answer

- No, I can't think of any.
- I don't know for sure.
- Yes, she does.

Growth History

출생, 성장에 대해 물어본다.

• Question

- Can you tell me about her birth history?
- How has her growth been till today?
- Can you tell me about her eating habits?

• Answer

- I fed her whole milk and solid food. I didn't breast-feed my child.
- She was growing very well.
- She was born at 40 weeks by vaginal delivery with no complications.

Dialogue

D: Good morning, Ms. Lee? Let me introduce myself. My name is Dr. Kim. I'm a doctor working on this hospital. I'm going to ask you some questions and do a physical exam on you. After that I'll discuss with you what I think so far.

P: OK.

D: If you have any questions, I'd be happy to answer them anytime. How old is he?

P: He is almost 1 year old.

D: How can I help you?

P: My son is having a high fever.

D: Ah··· You must be worried. when did the child temperature begin to rise?

P: I'm very concerned. It's been about a week.

D: How high was it?

P: It was 38.8 degrees when I measured it at home.

D: Was the temperature high the whole time?

P: Well. There's up and down but it's high most of the time.

D: Did you give him any fever reducer?

P: Yeah. He has taken some Tylenol, but I don't think it's working.

D: Was there any time his fever went over 41 degrees?

P: No, not that high.

D: Do you think he's sick any other than fever?

P: No, I'm not sure. He's just crying···

D: Is he sweating a lot?

P: Not really.

D: Are there any changes in his weight recently?

P: No.

D: Does he have some trouble breathing?

P: No, I don't think so.

D: Are there any noticeable rashes on his body?

P: No. There aren't.

D: Was there any vomiting? or changes in his stool?

P: No. There wasn't.

D: How about his urine? anything unusual?

P: No··· nothing special.

D: Has he been eating well lately?

P: Not good. He's not eating well since he had fever.

D: Does he sleep well at night?

P: No. He had to wake up a couple of times because of his fever.

D: Has he been getting his vaccinations regularly?

P: Yeah, since last month.

D: Does he have a record for any surgery or drug allergies?

P: No. He hasn't.

D: Does he go to any daycare centers?

P: Yes, he does.

D: Were there any other children there who had the same symptoms as him?

P: I'm not sure.

D: Is there any other family members who has fever?

P: No. Just my son.

D: Have you been traveling with him recently?

P: No.

D: Can you tell me about his birth history? How has his growth been till now?

P: He was born at 42 weeks by normal delivery with no complications.

D: Does your child have any congenital disorders?

P: Nope.

16. Weight Loss and Gain

Differential Diagnosis

	Diagnosis
Weight loss	Hyperthyroidism, cancer, dieting and diet drugs, anorexia nervosa, malabsorption, HIV infection
Weight gain	Hypothyroidism, Cushing's syndrome, polycystic ovary syndrome, diabetes melitus, smoking cessation, drug side effect, depression

Amount and Onset and Duration

체중 감소와 증가가 있었는지, 언제부터 있었는지, 체중 감소와 증가의 기간은 얼마나 되는지 등을 물어본다.

- Question
  - How many pounds did you gain and lose?
  - Have you noticed any change in your weight?
  - Since when have your weight been increased and decreased?
  - Over what period of time did it happen?
  - Was the weight gain and loss intentional?
- Answer
  - I have gained 20 pounds.
  - It started 3 months ago.
  - I don't feel like I'm losing weight. I'm not sure why mom is so worried.

Appetite

식욕에 변화가 있는지 물어본다.

• Question
  - How is your appetite?
  - Has there been any change in your appetite?

• Answer
  - I have a good appetite.

Diet History

식사 습관, 주로 식사하는 종류와 양에 대해 물어본다.

• Question
  - Has there been any change in your eating habits?
  - What do you usually eat?
  - Did you eat anything unusual lately?
  - What did you eat before the symptoms started?
  - Is there any kind of special diet that you are following?

• Answer
  - I eat lots of fruits and vegetables.
  - I stay away from fatty foods and high carbonates.
  - The usual. I haven't changed anything in my diet in more than 10 years.

Associated Symptoms

감별진단해야 할 Hyper and hypothyroidism, cancer, Cushing's syndrome 질환과 관련된 문진을 한다.

- Question
  - Have you ever been fatigued recently?
  - Do you have any problems falling asleep?
  - How many hours do you sleep?
  - How many bowel movements do you have in a day and week?
  - Have you noticed your heart pounding recently?
  - Have you grown any hair in your face, like a mustache or a beard?
- Answer
  - I'm tired all day. I have no energy.
  - I could sleep 20 hours a day if I did't have to work.
  - I move my bowels once a week.
  - No, I have not.

Past Medical History

- Question
  - Are you taking any medications?
  - Are you taking any over-the-counter drugs, vitamins, or herbs?
  - Do you have any other medical problems?
- Answer
  - I have bipolar disorder.
  - I was started on lithium 6 months ago.
  - I haven't had any problems since then.

OB and GYN History

여성의 경우 임신에 의해 체중이 증가했을 수 있으므로 이에 대해 물어보고, hyper와 hypothyroidism 시에 체중 변화와 함께 menstruation의 변화가 있을 수 있으므로 이에 대해 문진한다.

- Question
  - How often do you get your menstrual period?
  - When was the first day of your last menstrual period?
  - How many pads or tampons do you use per day?
  - Have you noticed any change in your periods or amounts?
  - Is there any possibility of your pregnancy?
- Answer
  - I used to get my period every four weeks, but recently I've been getting it every six weeks or more. The period lasts seven days.
  - It was 2~3 a day, but the blood flow is becoming less, and I use only one a day now.
  - I didn't menstruate for 3 months.
  - I didn't have any sexual relationships nowadays, because I'm too busy.

Psychiatric History

Body image, anxiety, depression 등에 대한 현재 상황에 문진과 함께, 이전 정신과적 질환으로 진단받고 medication 중인지 여부를 질문한다.

- Question
  - Do you take interest or pleasure in your daily activities?
  - Do you have difficulty concentrating?
  - Has anyone in your family ever been experienced depression?
  - Can you still perform your daily functions or activities?

Social History

- Question
  - Do you smoke? If yes, how long have you smoked?
  - Did you quit smoking recently?
  - Do you have a lot of stressful situations on your job?
  - Tell me about your use of alcohol.
- Answer
  - I quit smoking 3 months ago. I had smoked 2 packs a day for 10 years.

Familial History

- Question
  - Does anyone in your family have any particular disease?
  - Do you have a family history of thyroid disease?
  - Is there any obese person in your family?
- Answer
  - My younger sister has a thyroid problem and takes pills for it.
  - My mother and sister are obese.

Dialogue

D: Good morning, Ms. Lee?

P: Good morning.

D: Let me introduce myself. My name is Dr. Kim. I'm a doctor working on this hospital. I'm going to ask you some questions and do a physical exam on you. After that I'll discuss with you what I think so far. If you have any questions, I'd be happy to answer them anytime.

P: OK.

D: What brought you in here today?

P: I'm getting thin even though I eat a lot. I'm really worried about my health.

D: How many kilograms did you lose?

P: I have lost 7 kilograms.

D: Over what period of time did it happen?

P: Over 6 months.

D: Is there any change in your diet?

P: No, I eat usual meal. I haven't changed anything in my diet.

D: Recently, you've exercised more than usual?

P: No, I haven't.

D: Have you ever been fatigued recently?

P: I'm tired all day. I have no energy.

D: Have you noticed your heart pounding recently?

P: Yes, even when I relax, there is a pounding.

D: Do you have a hard time adjusting to hot temperature?

P: Yes, I can't stand the heat. And I sweat a lot.

D: Do you have any change in your bowel movements?

P: Yes, I have diarrhea.

D: Do you take any medications?

P: No, nothing.

D: Have you ever been hospitalized?

P: No, I have not.

D: Has anyone in the family ever been diagnosed with thyroid disease?

P: My sister had diagnosed with thyroid cancer, so she had surgery.

D: Well, thank you for your cooperation Ms. Lee. Now we're going to do a physical exam on you. I know that you're not well so I'll be as gentle as possible. Let me wash my hands first.

P: OK…

D: Ms. Lee. I need to examine your thyroid, it's the hormone gland in your neck area. First let me take a look at your gland.

D: I need to touch your neck gland. Now I need you to swallow for me while I touch your neck from your back. Would you like a glass of tap water so that you can swallow more easily?

P: Yes, please.

D: OK. Here you are. Please take a drink and please swallow when I tell you to.

P: OK.

D: Swallow… swallow… OK. Well, thank you for your cooperation Ms. Lee. Let me tell you what I think so far.

D: Based on the informations you gave me, the most likely diagnosis is what we call graves disease which means that your thyroid works too much.

P: Oh, then how it can be treated?

D: First, we have to do more exams to make sure the diagnosis. And then, if it is what we thought, I'll control the thyroid function with medications.

P: OK.

D: Well, I think we're all done here. I'll meet you at tomorrow to discuss the results with you. Until then, please take care. Bye.

17. Upper GI Bleeding

Differential Diagnosis

1. Bleeding peptic ulcer
2. Gastritis
3. Gastric cancer
4. Esophageal varices
5. Mallory-Weiss tear

Onset and Duration

- Question
  - When did it start?
  - When it comes, how long does it last?
- Answer
  - It was started at 7 A.M.
  - It lasted about 5 minutes.
  - It is continuously bleeding 1 hour ago.

Context

심한 구토, 알코올 섭취, 코피가 난 후 상황에 대해 물어본다.

- Question
  - After you vomited, did you feel light-headedness?
  - Did you drink alcohol before you vomited out?
  - Was nosebleed accompanied with?

• Answer

- I felt light-headed.
- I haven't drunken since I was diagnosed with liver cirrhosis.

Nature

구체적 증상과 정도에 대해 물어본다.

• Question

- Was brownish, blackish or reddish?
- How much was the vomitus? A teaspoon? Two teaspoons? A cupful?

• Answer

- It was a cup of reddish blood.

• Duration

- When it comes how long does it last?

• Context

After severe vomiting, alcohol ingestion, nosebleed

- After you vomited, did you feel light-headedness?
- Did you drink alcohol before you vomited out?
- Was nosebleed accompanied with?

Associated Symptoms

관련증상(메스꺼움, 복통, 소화불량)을 물어본다.

• Question

- Do you have abdominal pain?
- Do you feel nausea before vomiting?

- Do you have problem with digestion?

- Answer
  - Yes, I feel my abdomen is distended.
  - Yes, I'm nauseous before vomiting.
  - Yes, I think I can't digest fatty foods.

Past History

과거력(위궤양 질환, 간 질환, 복부 대동맥류의 혈관내 치료, 출혈 경향)을 물어본다.

- Question
  - Have you ever had abdominal aortic aneurysm repair surgery?
  - Have you ever been diagnosed with peptic ulcer disease or liver disease?
  - Have you ever been diagnosed with easy bleeding?
- Answer
  - None.
  - Yes. I heard I am HBV carrier.
  - Well. Recently, I have noticed that I am bruised easy.

Social History

약물 치료 중인지 (특히 Warfarin, NSAIDs) 여부를 물어본다.

- Question
  - Are you taking any kind of drugs like warfarin or NSAIDs?
- Answer
  - Doctor diagnosed me as Osteoarthritis, so I have taken NSAID for 3 years.

18. Blood in Stool

Differential Diagnosis

- Lower GI bleeding
  - Colorectal cancer
  - Hemorrhoids
  - Diverticulosis
  - Angiodysplasia
  - Pseudomembranous colitis
  - Ulcerative colitis
  - Crohn's disease
- Upper GI bleeding

Onset

- Question
  - When did it start?
  - How long has it lasted?
- Answer
  - It started 1 month ago.
  - I saw some blood mixed in with the stool last Monday.

Nature

- Question
  - Can you describe the color of stools?
  - Were there any black tarry stools or red blood in the stools?
  - How much does the blood in the stools?
- Answer
  - It was bright red.
  - It was about a spoon of blood.

Associated Symptoms

- Question
  - Do you have pain?
  - Do you think the stools remain even though you have passed them out?
  - Do you have constipation?
  - Do you have diarrhea?
- Answer
  - No, I don't have pain.
  - Yes, a little.
  - Well, I have had constipation for a long time, and I keep taking laxatives. At first I used to get some relief, but now there is no benefit from them.
  - I have a diarrhea for the past 2 days.

Past History

- Question
  - Did you have trauma on your bowel or rectal area by accident, recently?
  - Have you ever had this before?
  - Have you ever had colonoscopy?
  - Did you ever been diagnosed with atherosclerotic vascular disease?
- Answer
  - No, I don't have any trauma.
  - No, this is the first event.
  - Yes, I had colonoscopy in regular health check ups.
  - No, I didn't have diagnosed any vascular disease.

Social History

- Question
  - Are you taking any kind of drugs like Warfarin?
- Answer
  - No, I'm not taking any drugs except vitamins.

Dialogue

D: Good morning, Mr. Lee?

P: Good morning.

D: Let me introduce myself. My name is Dr. Kim. I'm a doctor working on this hospital. I'm going to ask you some questions and do a physical exam on you. After that, I'll discuss with you what I think so far.

P: OK.

D: If you have any questions, I'd be happy to answer them anytime. What seems to be your problem?

P: I vomited blood.

D: Oh, you must be very surprised. When did you vomit blood?

P: Yesterday. I was surprised a lot.

D: Was it the first time?

P: Yes, I've never vomited blood before.

D: Can you tell me about the color? Was it bright red, or dark brown?

P: It was bright red.

D: Can you tell me more details about the situation?

P: I had my birthday party yesterday. I had to drink too much. Actually I'm a poor drinker. So I vomited many times, and vomited blood in the end.

D: Did you have bowel movements after the event?

P: Yes, this morning I had.

D: Then what was your stool color?

P: It was very dark like coke.

D: Are you dizzy now?

P: No, I'm not.

D: Have you noticed any shortness of breath?

P: No, I haven't.

D: Have you ever been diagnosed with peptic ulcer disease or liver disease?

P: No, I've never. I've been very healthy.

D: OK. Do you take any medications?

P: Just multivitamins.

D: Have you ever smoked?

P: No, I haven't.

D: Do you drink alcohol frequently?

P: Well, I drink about once in a week.

D: How much you drink?

P: I usually drink 3 or 4 glasses of beer.

D: Well, thank you for your cooperation Mr. Lee. Now we're going to do a physical exam on you. I know that you're not well so I'll be as gentle as possible. Let me wash my hands first.

P: OK.

D: Let me look at your eyes. If you have severe bleeding, your conjunctiva would be pale. But fortunately, it is OK.

D: Let me take a look at your stomach area.

D: OK. Now I need to listen to your belly. Well, your bowel sound is normal.

D: Now I'm going to tap on your belly. If it hurts, please let me know.

D: I'm going to press lightly on your stomach area. Tell me if it hurts.

D: Now I'm going to press a little more deeply. Please tell me if it hurts.

D: Now, I have to check your anus with my finger. I know it heard awkward, but it is very important to confirm whether the bleeding stops or not. So could you permit to do?

P: Well, OK.

D: Well, thank you for your cooperation Mr. Lee. Let me tell you what I think so far.

P: OK.

D: Based on the informations you gave me, the most likely diagnosis is what we call mallory weiss syndrome which means that your esophagus tears.

P: Oh, is it a severe disease?

D: Well, if you have severe bleeding, it will be a problem. But fortunately, in your case, it doesn't look severe. So, don't worry too much.

P: Oh, thanks god.

D: But we have to do some exams including endoscope. If you have active bleeding, I will treat it with endoscope. OK?

P: OK.

D: Well, I think we're all done here. I'll meet you at tomorrow to endoscope and discuss the results with you. Until then, please take care. Bye.

19. Constipation and Diarrhea

Differential Diagnosis

Constipation	Diarrhea
Colorectal cancer Low-fat diet Irritable bowel syndrome Substance abuse (e.g., heroin) Depression Hypothyroidism	Infectious diarrhea Food poisoning Inflammatory bowel disease Pseudomembranous colitis Traveler's diarrhea Hyperthyroidism Lactose intolerance Celiac disease

Onset and Duration

- Question
  - How long did you notice any change in your bowel movements?
- Answer
  - I noticed that 1 month ago.
  - It started yesterday at 2 P.M.

Nature

- Question
  - How often does it come?
  - Do you have any difficulties?
  - What does the stool look like in terms of bulk?
- Answer
  - I have about 6 bowel movements per day.
  - Yes, it is struggle for me to start.
  - It was watery and large amounts.

Associated Symptoms

- Question
  - Do you have pain?
  - During passage of stool, is it hard and perhaps painful?
  - Do you feel your bowel distended?
  - Do you think the stools remain even though you have passed them out?
  - Can you describe the color of stools?
  - Were there any black tarry stools or reddish stools?
- Answer
  - No, I don't have pain.
  - No, I don't feel like that.
  - It was brown color.
  - Yes, a little blood in stool.

Accompanying Symptoms

- Question
  - Do you have a hard time adjusting to hot or cold temperature?
  - Have you noticed your heart pounding recently?
  - Do you noticed any swellings in your body?
  - Do you feel tired than usual these days?
  - Do you feel sad?
- Answer
  - No, I don't have.

Past History

- Question
  - Have you ever had any kind of abdominal surgeries?
  - Have you ever been diagnosed with high blood sugar?
  - Have you ever been diagnosed with pancreatitis?
- Answer
  - I had appendectomy 2 years ago.
  - No, I don't have.

Social History 1

- Question
  - Do you enjoy low fiber diet?
  - Do you like fatty food?
  - Are you taking any antibiotics?
  - Did you contact with people with diarrhea, recently?
  - Did you travel, recently?
- Answer
  - Yes, I usually eat meat.
  - No, I don't take any antibiotics.
  - My roommate have diarrhea, recently.

Social History 2

- Question
  - Are you sexually active?
  - How many partners do you have?
  - What are your sexual preferences? Male? Female? Or both?

- Do you use any contraceptive methods?
- Have you ever been diagnosed with any kind of sexual transmitted disease including HIV?
- Have you ever used tobacco in any form?
- Do you drink alcohol?
- How much? How long?

Family History

- Question
  - Has anyone in the family ever been diagnosed with colon cancer?
- Answer
  - My grandfather died for colon cancer.
  - My parents are alive and in good health.

Dialogue

D: Good morning, Ms. Lee?

P: Good morning.

D: Let me introduce myself. My name is Dr. Kim. I'm a doctor working on this hospital. I'm going to ask you some questions and do a physical exam on you. After that I'll discuss with you what I think so far.

P: OK.

D: If you have any questions, I'd be happy to answer them anytime. What brings you here today?

P: I have diarrhea.

D: How long did you notice any change in your bowel movements?

P: I noticed that 6 months ago.

D: Can you describe to me how the stool looks like?

P: It is loose and brown.

D: What does it look like in terms of bulk?

P: It isn't large amount, but I have about 7 bowel movements per day.

D: Is there any change in your body weight?

P: No.

D: Do you have abdominal pain?

P: Yes, I have.

D: Can you tell me exactly where it hurts?

P: Right here. Around the navel.

D: Then, is there anything that makes it better?

P: Yes, after movements, it gets better.

D: Besides the diarrhea, do you have constipation?

P: Yes, I have.

D: Is there any change in your diet?

P: No, I eat usual meal.

D: Have you ever had any kind of abdominal surgeries?

P: No, I haven't.

D: Have you ever smoked?

P: No, I haven't.

D: Do you drink alcohol?

P: No, I don't.

D: Has anyone in the family ever been diagnosed with colon cancer?

P: Yes, my grandfather passed away with colon cancer.

D: Oh, I'm sorry. Well, thank you for your cooperation Mr. Lee. Now we're going to do a physical exam on you. I know that you're not well, so I'll be as gentle as possible. Let me wash my hands first.

P: OK.

D: Let me take a look at your stomach area. I notice that you have a very big mole here.

P: Oh, I've had that since I was little. Nothing important.

D: OK. Now I need to listen to your belly. Well, your bowel sound is normal. Now I'm going to tap on your belly. If it hurts, please let me know. I'm going to press lightly on your stomach area. Tell me if it hurts. Now I'm going to press a little more deeply. Please tell me if it hurts. Well, thank you for your cooperation Mr. Lee. Let me tell you what I think so far.

P: OK.

D: Based on the informations you gave me, the most likely diagnosis is what we call irritable bowel syndrome which means that your bowel is very sensitive.

P: Oh, is it a severe disease?

D: No, it isn't. But in case you have a severe disease, we have to do some more exams. They're just for making it sure that you are OK, so don't worry. OK?

P: OK.

D: Well, I think we're all done here. I'll meet you at tomorrow to discuss the results with you. Until then, please take care. Bye.

지은이 소개

이종호 교수

한림의과대학 졸업

현재 한림대학교 의과대학 교수(약리학)

한림의료관광인재양성센터 국제의사팀장

안무업 교수

원주의과대학 졸업

현재 한림대학교 의과대학 교수(응급의학)

한림대학교 춘천성심병원 응급센터장

국제 진료 영어

초판 발행 2011년 3월 22일

지은이 이종호 · 안무업
펴낸이 고화숙
펴낸곳 도서출판 소화
등록 제13-412호
주소 서울시 영등포구 영등포동 7가 94-97
전화 02-2677-5890
팩스 02-2636-6393
홈페이지 www.sowha.com

ISBN 978-89-8410-403-7 93740

값 15,000원